Mediterranean Easy Cookbook

A Full Collection of Tasty Leek, Beetroot & Avocado Mediterranean Recipes

Alex Brawn

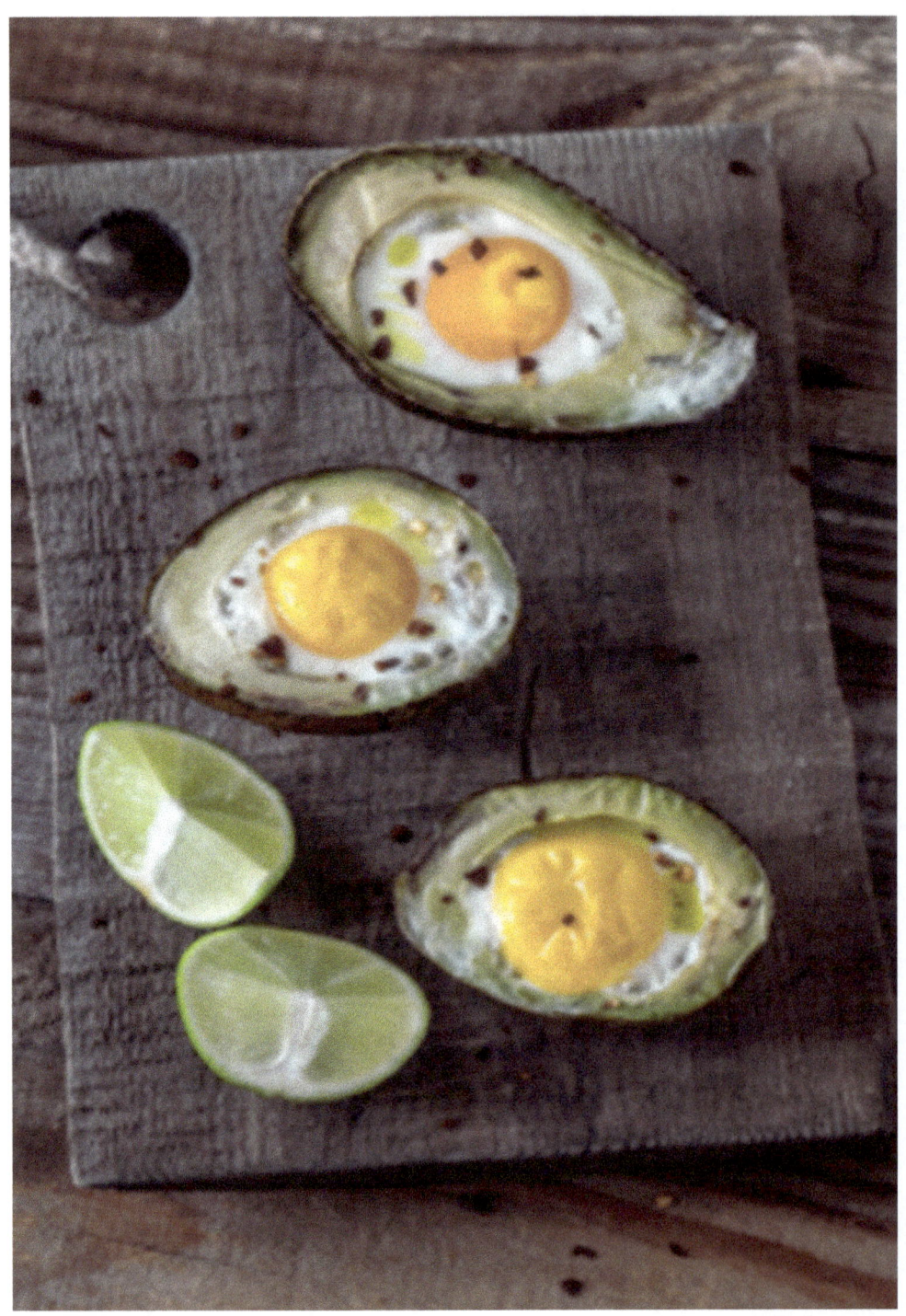

Table of Contents

5

Crostini of smoked salmon butter and poached leeks

Ingredients

- 5 sprigs of fresh chervil
- 160g of unsalted butter
- 200ml of white wine
- 10 baby leeks
- 130g of smoked salmon
- 60g of unsalted butter
- 60ml of olive oil
- 20ml of fresh lemon juice
- 2 fresh bay leaves
- 12 slices of ciabatta
- 3 sprigs of fresh thyme
- 200ml of quality fish stock
- 40g of salted baby capers

Directions

- Combine the butter with smoked salmon, and lemon juice in a food processor, blend until smooth.
- Season and set aside.

- Combine butter, olive oil, bay leaves, and thyme to a wide, shallow saucepan over a medium-low heat, let simmer.
- Add the leeks, let cook for 10 minutes, until golden.
- Pour in the stock with the wine, cover with a baking paper, let cook for 15 minutes.
- Remove from the heat and rest the leeks in the liquid.
- Put the capers in a small saucepan with enough olive oil to cover.
- Place over a high heat, fry until the capers crisp up.
- Transfer the capers to a plate lined with kitchen paper using a slotted spoon.
- Heat a griddle pan over medium high heat.
- Brush the ciabatta with olive oil and toast until golden.
- Spread the toasted ciabatta generously with the smoked salmon butter.
- Serve and enjoy topped with the leeks and fried capers

Ham and leek quiche

Ingredients

- 300ml of semi-skimmed milk
- 2 leeks
- 1 shallot
- 8 sprigs of fresh thyme
- 4 sheets of filo pastry
- 75g of mature Cheddar
- 60g of smoked ham
- 3 large eggs
- 10g of unsalted butter
- 200g of sprouting broccoli
- 1 tablespoon of olive oil

Directions

- Preheat the oven to 350°F.
- Melt butter in a pan, then sauté the leeks with the shallot and half the thyme leaves for 5 minutes.
- Blanch the broccoli in boiling salted water for about 3 minutes. Drain.

- Brush a quiche tin with a little of the olive oil, drape with a layer of filo pastry, leaving some overhanging.
- Brush the filo with a little more oil.
- Scatter over some of the remaining thyme leaves and layer another piece of filo on top. Repeat layering the oil, thyme and filo until you have a fully lined quiche base.
- Bake the case for 5 minutes.
- Stir the broccoli together with the smoked ham through the leek mixture.
- Spoon the filling over the pastry base.
- Beat the eggs with milk and a pinch of black pepper, grate in cheese.
- Pour over the vegetables and ham.
- Place grate over the rest of the cheese.
- Place the baking tray, let bake for 30 minutes.
- Let rest for 15 minutes, serve and enjoy.

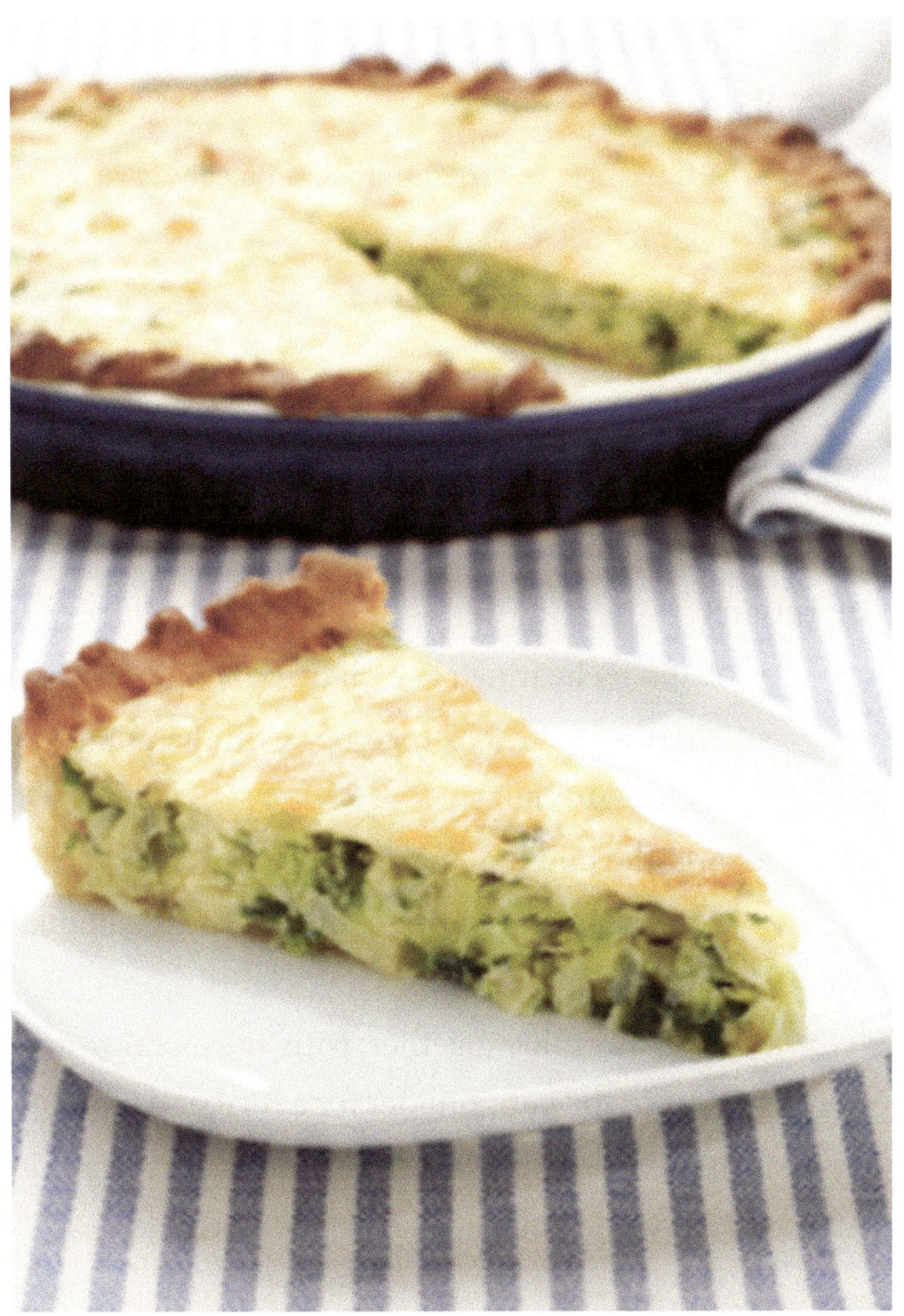

Leek, potato, and pea soup

Ingredients

- A few sprigs of fresh flat-leaf parsley
- 2 large leeks
- 200g of frozen peas
- 1 large potato
- 1½ tablespoons of olive oil
- 1 teaspoon of bouillon powder
- 400ml of milk

Directions

- Begin by heating olive oil over medium heat.
- Then, add the leek together with the potatoes, fry for 5 minutes.
- Add the bouillon powder.
- Pour in 400ml water, reduce the heat, simmer for 10 minutes.
- Add the milk together with the parsley and peas to the pan, simmer for a further 5 minutes to warm through.
- Serve and enjoy.

Chickpea, leek, and carrot stew

Ingredients

- ½ tablespoon of olive oil
- 1 small leek
- 1 small carrot
- 2 tablespoons of natural yoghurt
- 1 x 210g tin of chickpeas

Directions

- Heat olive oil in a medium pan over medium heat.
- Add the leek, let cook until softened, then add the carrots with 200ml water.
- Bring to the boil, when covered, then reduce to a simmer for until the vegetables are tender.
- Drain, then add the chickpeas, let warm through for 5 minutes, then remove.
- Let cool briefly, then stir through the yoghurt.
- Mash until fairly smooth, with some soft lumps.
- Serve and enjoy.

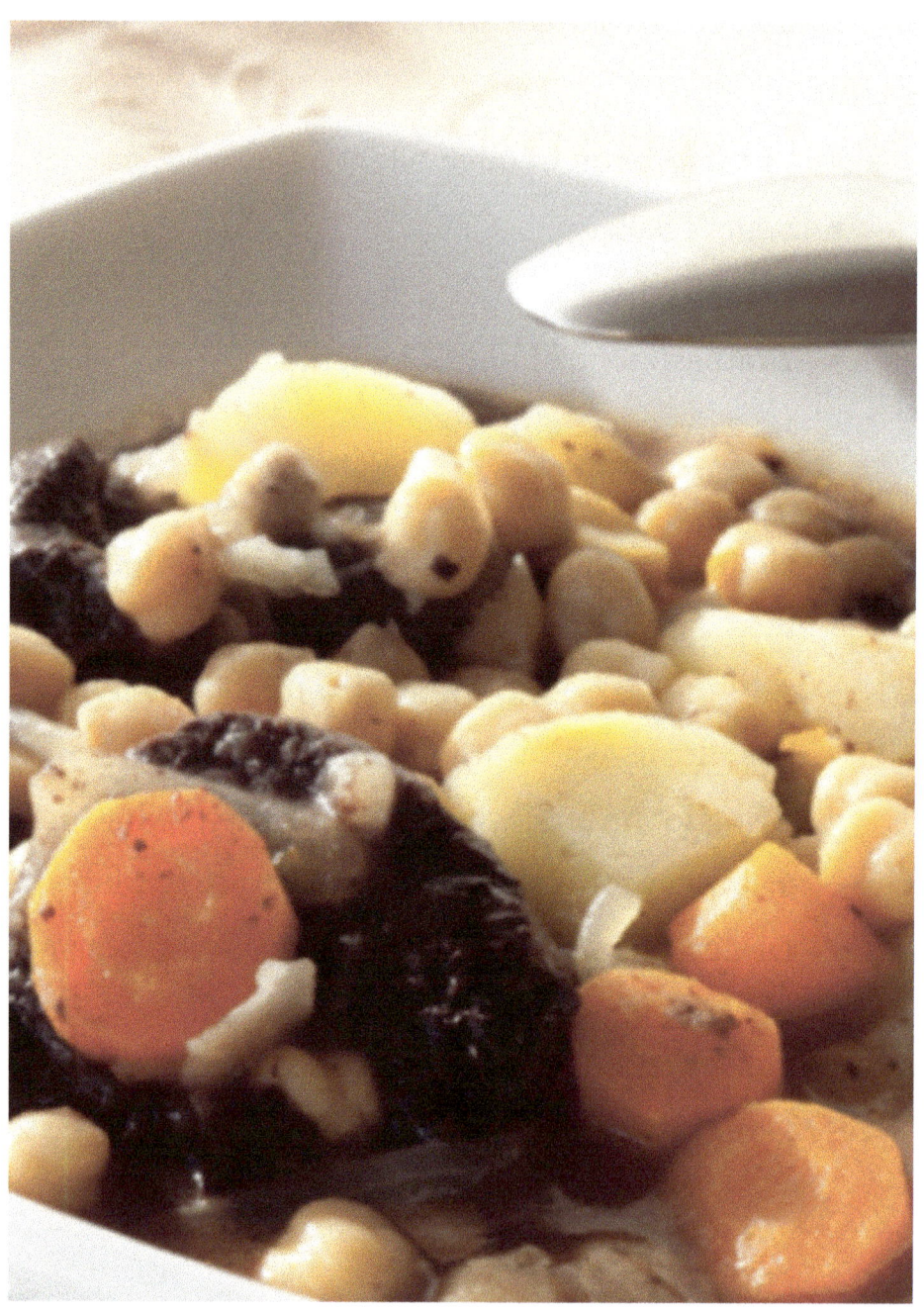

Chicken, leek, and pea pasta bake

Ingredients

- 200g of cooked chicken
- 1 tablespoon butter
- 225ml of milk
- 150g of frozen peas
- 350g of pasta
- 250g of ricotta cheese
- Olive oil
- 2 leeks
- 2 cloves of garlic
- 60g of Parmesan cheese
- 100ml of chicken stock
- 100ml of white wine

Directions

- Preheat the oven to 350°F and grease your baking dish.
- Then, cook the pasta in a large pan of boiling salted water, let be undercooked.
- Drain any excess water.

- Return to the saucepan and coat with a drizzle of olive oil.
- Place butter in a frying pan, fry the leeks for 10 minutes.
- Add the garlic, stock, and wine and cook for 10 minutes.
- Add the peas, cook for 30 seconds, stirring once.
- Add the leek mixture, chicken, milk, and 2/3 of the ricotta to the drained pasta.
- Let combine.
- Season with salt and pepper.
- Spoon the pasta mixture into the baking dish.
- Top with the remaining ricotta, grate over the Parmesan, and drizzle with olive oil.
- Bake for 25 minutes.
- Serve and enjoy.

Sweet leek, ricotta, and tomato lasagna

Ingredients

- 1 packet of lasagna sheets
- 4 leeks, thinly sliced
- 75g of fresh parmesan, grated
- 2 red onions, thinly sliced
- Sea salt
- 250g of spinach
- Olive oil
- 350g of ricotta
- Freshly ground black pepper
- 1-liter tomato sauce
- 125g of mozzarella ball

Directions

- Preheat your oven ready to 350°F.
- Heat a large saucepan, add a splash of olive oil when hot.
- Add the leeks together with the sliced red onions, and sweat, for 10 minutes.
- Add the chopped spinach and briefly cook until wilted down.

- Drain off any excess.
- Mix the ricotta into the leek and onion mixture.
- Season with a tiny pinch of salt and pepper.
- Spoon a quarter of the tomato sauce into the bottom of 6 individual ovenproof dishes.
- Cover with sheets of lasagna.
- Then, spread half the leek and ricotta mixture over the lasagna.
- Add the remaining tomato sauce. Repeat with all the lasagna sheets, leek and ricotta mixture, and the remaining tomato sauce.
- But finish with a layer of lasagna sheets.
- Tear the mozzarella into small pieces and dot over the top of the lasagna.
- Sprinkle with the Parmesan.
- Bake the individual lasagna for 30 minutes.
- Serve and enjoy.

Sausages with pan cooked chutney and leek mash

Ingredients

- 5cm piece of fresh ginger, grated
- 1kg of potatoes, peeled and halved
- 3 tablespoons of balsamic vinegar
- Olive oil
- 2.5cm piece cinnamon stick
- 2 leeks, sliced
- 1 handful of fresh cranberries
- 2 red onions, cut into thin wedges
- 8 pork sausages
- 200ml of milk
- Extra virgin olive oil
- 1 sprig fresh sage, leaves picked

Directions

- Begin by cooking the potatoes in simmering water for 15 minutes.
- Drain, cover and set aside.
- Add olive of oil to a separate saucepan with the leeks.

- Sweat gently for about 5 minutes.
- Then, add bring to the boil the milk.
- Turn off the heat, then add to the potatoes.
- Mash and season to taste. Cover and set aside.
- Preheat the grill to medium.
- Add a splash of olive oil to a frying pan over a medium heat.
- Fry the sage leaves until crisp, set aside.
- Sauté the onions for 5 minutes, add the cranberries together with the cinnamon and a splash of water.
- Let simmer for 15 minutes, stirring, until the onions are soft.
- Add the ginger together with the vinegar, cook for 30 seconds. Season.
- Place the sausages under the grill for 15 minutes, turning frequently, until cooked.
- Serve and enjoy with the chutney, mash, and sage leaves.

Slow roasted balsamic tomatoes with baby leeks and basil

Ingredients

- 12 plum tomatoes
- 200ml of balsamic vinegar
- 4 cloves garlic
- 2 tablespoons of extra virgin olive oil
- Freshly ground black pepper
- 1 handful of fresh basil
- 12 fresh bay leaves
- 12 baby leeks
- Sea salt

Directions

- Preheat the oven to 325°F.
- Score the tops of the tomatoes with a cross.
- Take an earthenware dish that the tomatoes will fit snugly into.
- Sprinkle the garlic and basil all over the bottom.
- Stand the tomatoes next to each other in the tray, on top of the garlic and basil, then push

the bay leaves well into the scores in the tomatoes, season.

- Lay the leeks on a board.
- Sprinkle generously with salt and pepper.
- Squeeze the seasoning into the mixture by pressing with a rolling pin.
- Weave the leeks in and around the tomatoes.
- Pour over the balsamic vinegar, drizzle over the olive oil.
- Let bake in the preheated oven for 1 hour.
- Remove the bay leaves.
- Serve and enjoy over pasta.

Roasted concertina squid with grilled leeks and a warm chorizo dressing

Ingredients

- 4 medium-sized squid
- Extra virgin olive oil
- 100g of chorizo sausage
- 2 cloves garlic
- 8 baby leeks
- 3 tablespoons of balsamic vinegar
- Olive oil
- Juice from one lime
- 1 sprig fresh rosemary
- 2 lemons, halved
- Sea salt
- Freshly ground black pepper
- 1 bulb fennel
- 1 radicchio, leaves separated

Directions

- Firstly, preheat a griddle pan.
- Then, preheat your oven ready to 475°F.

- Parboil the baby leeks for 3 minutes in a pan of boiling salted water.
- Drain in a colander, then let steam dry.
- Dress with some olive oil and a pinch of sea salt.
- Griddle, and cook the leek until marked with the griddle lining, add the fennel wedges, chargrill these dry on both sides until they are also marked.
- Add the radicchio leaves and dry grill to wilt.
- Put the leeks fennel and radicchio into a large bowl.
- Heat a frying pan with olive oil.
- Fry the chorizo until the fat renders out, then add the rosemary with the garlic, toss briefly and remove.
- Add the balsamic vinegar with some lemon juice to the pan, mix.
- Drizzle some olive oil over each squid, sprinkle with some salt and pepper, toss.

- Preheat an ovenproof pan with bit of olive oil, toss the reserved tentacles in the oil for 1 minute.
- Add all the squid and whack the pan in the preheated oven briefly until cooked.
- Pour the chorizo dressing over your chargrilled veggies with a squeeze of lemon juice.
- Serve and enjoy.

Roasted baby leek with thyme

Ingredients

- 2 cloves garlic
- 20 baby leeks
- 1 teaspoon of chopped fresh thyme leaves
- Olive oil
- Red wine vinegar

Directions

- Preheat your oven ready to 400°F.
- Place the leeks in a pan of boiling salted water for 3 minutes.
- Drain any excess water.
- Toss with olive oil, chopped thyme leaves, a splash of red wine vinegar, and the garlic in a bowl.
- Arrange the leeks in one layer in a baking tray.
- Let roast in the preheated oven for 10 minutes or so until golden.
- Serve and enjoy.

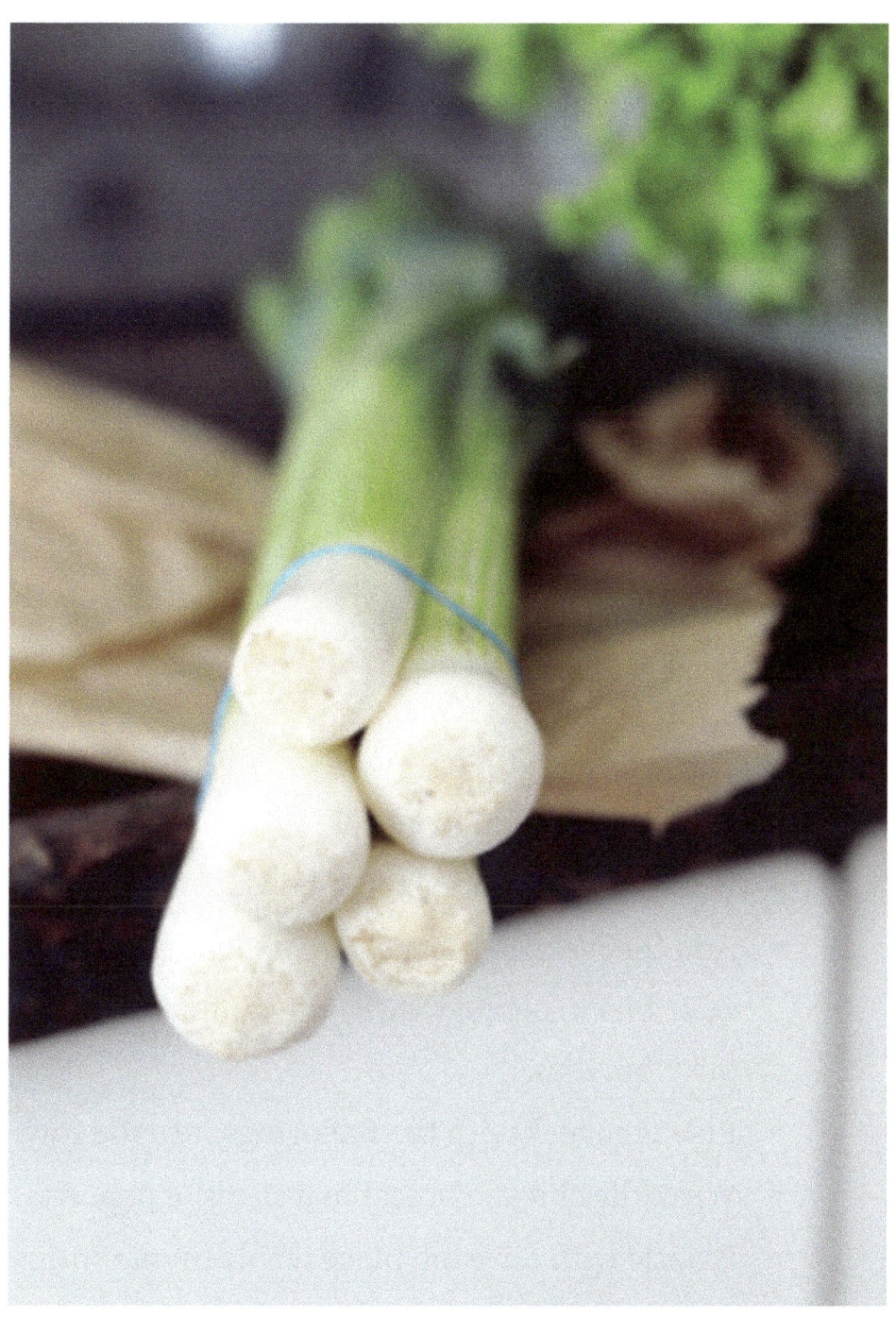

Roasted chicken breast with pancetta, leeks, and thyme

Ingredients

- Olive oil
- 1 chicken breast
- 1 pinch of sea salt
- 2 whole sprigs thyme
- 1 pinch of freshly ground black pepper
- 1 large leek
- 1 small swig of white wine
- 4 slices of pancetta

Directions

- Preheat the oven to 400°F.
- Place 1 chicken breast in a bowl.
- Add the leek, leek leaves, fresh thyme, pinch of salt, black pepper, swig of white wine, and olive oil, toss.
- Place the leek with the flavorings into the tray.
- Wrap the chicken breast in 4 slices of pancetta.
- Drizzle with olive oil, place whole thyme sprigs on top.

- Let cook for 35 minutes in the preheated.

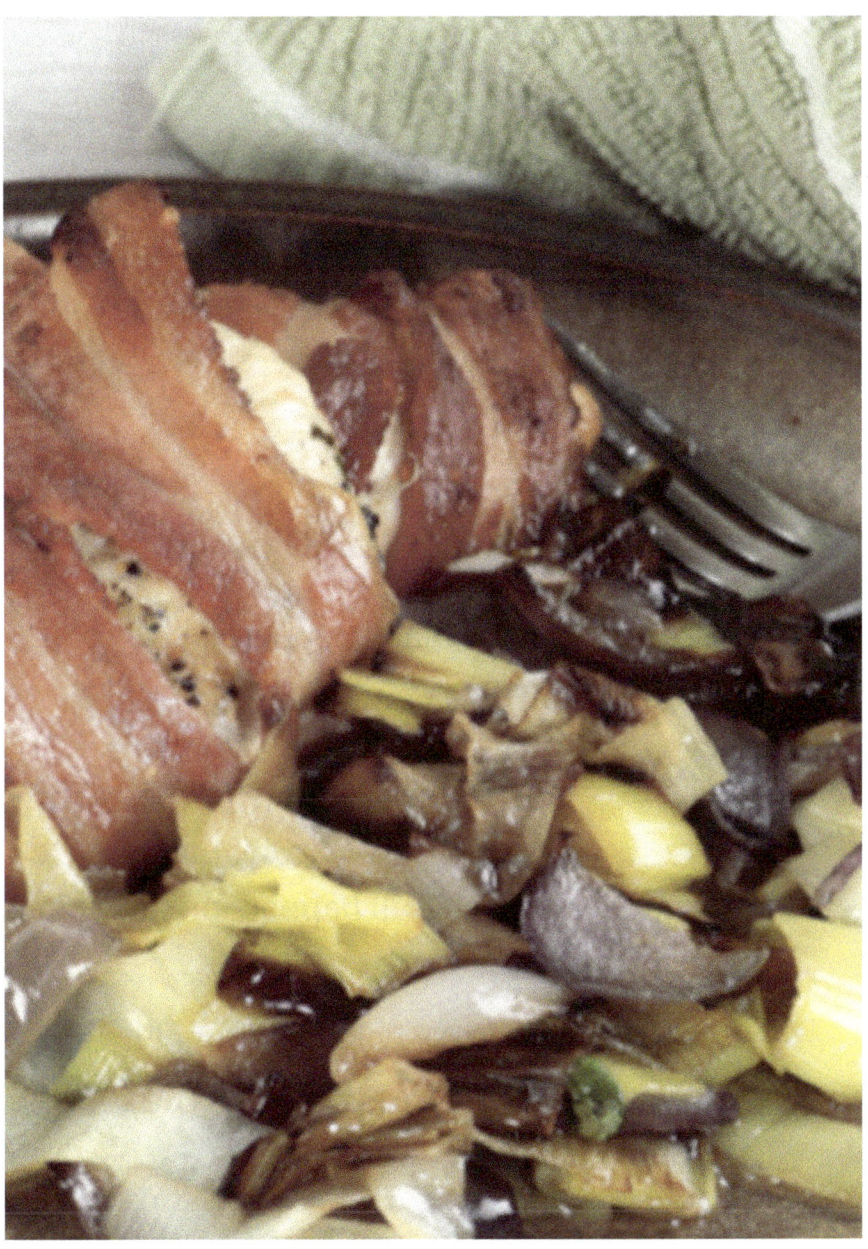

Chargrilled marinated vegetables

Ingredients

- 2 red peppers
- 1 clove garlic
- 1 large bunch of fresh basil
- 2 tablespoons of herb
- 2 yellow peppers
- 2 medium courgettes
- 1 bulb fennel
- 1 aubergine
- 8 baby leeks
- Freshly ground black pepper
- Sea salt
- Extra virgin olive oil

Directions

- Griddle pan, place all peppers on until black on all sides.
- Grill the courgette with the fennel together for 1 minute on each side.
- Transfer to a clean tea towel in one layer.

- Chargrill the aubergine slices, turn 4 times until marked.
- Transfer to the tea towel.
- Boil the baby leeks in salted water until cooked.
- Drain, then rub with bit of olive oil, and chargrill until lightly marked.
- Place all the vegetables into a large bowl.
- Bash some basil leaves in a pestle and mortar with a pinch of seasoning until a smooth pulp.
- Add about 8 tablespoons of extra virgin olive oil with vinegar.
- Pour over the vegetables and toss to coat in the basil oil. Discard the remaining basil leaves.
- Add sliced garlic to the bowl with the fennel tops.
- Give everything a good mix.
- Serve and enjoy.

Grilled fillet steak with the creamiest white beans and leeks

Ingredients

- 4 x 200g of fillet steaks
- 4 leeks
- 1 lemon
- Sea salt
- 1 small bunch of fresh thyme
- 2 cloves garlic
- Olive oil
- 1 small wineglass white wine
- Freshly ground black pepper
- 500g of tinned butter beans
- Peppery extra virgin olive oil
- 1 small handful freshly picked parsley leaves
- 1 tablespoon of fat-free natural yoghurt

Directions

- Firstly, sweat the leeks together with the thyme and garlic in a saucepan with a splash of olive oil over low heat for 20 minutes.
- Raise the heat, then add the white wine.

- Let the wine come to the boil.
- After which add the beans with a splash of water, just to almost cover the beans.
- Let simmer for 10 minutes until the beans are creamy.
- Add the parsley together with the yoghurt and extra virgin olive oil.
- Taste, and adjust the seasoning.
- Heat a griddle pan until hot, season the steaks and pat with olive oil.
- Grill a steak for 3 minutes on each side for medium-rare.
- Remove from the grill on to a dish, let rest for 5 minutes.
- Squeeze over some lemon juice and drizzle with extra virgin olive oil.
- Carve the steaks into thick slices.
- Divide the creamy beans between plates and place the steak on top
- Serve and enjoy drizzled with resting juices.

Gravadlax recipe

Ingredients

- 50g of fresh grated horseradish
- 1 big bunch of fresh dill
- 200g of raw beets
- 1 lemon
- 100g of rock salt
- 50g of demerara sugar
- 1 x 700g side of salmon
- 50ml of vodka

Directions

- Place the beets in a food processor together with sugar, vodka, salt, and dill.
- Grate in the lemon zest and add horseradish, blend to combine.
- Rub bit of the mixture on to the salmon skin, then put on a large tray, skin side down, cover completely with the mixture.
- Cover the tray tightly with Clingfilm with a weight on top.
- Place into the fridge for 36 hours.

- Once cured, unwrap the fish, pour the juices down the sink and rub salty topping.
- Pat the fillet dry, then tightly wrap in Clingfilm. Keep in the fridge until needed.
- Slice and enjoy.

Beetroot, carrot, and orange salad

Ingredients

- ½ a bunch of fresh coriander
- Olive oil
- 2 oranges
- 500g of raw beetroot
- 1 tablespoon of sesame seeds
- 750g of carrots
- Extra virgin olive oil

Directions

- Preheat the oven to 400°F.
- Parboil the carrots in a large pan of boiling salted water for 5 minutes.
- Move to a colander using a slotted spoon.
- Place in the beets and parboil for 5 minutes, then drain.
- Transfer the carrots with the beets to a large roasting tin, then, drizzle with olive oil.
- Season with sea salt and black pepper.
- Let roast for 40 minutes, or until shiny, shake the tray occasionally.

- Toast the sesame seeds over low heat until golden, tossing regularly.
- Let cool, toss with the orange zest and segments, extra virgin olive oil.
- Arrange over a large platter, scatter over the toasted sesame seeds and coriander leaves.
- Serve and enjoy.

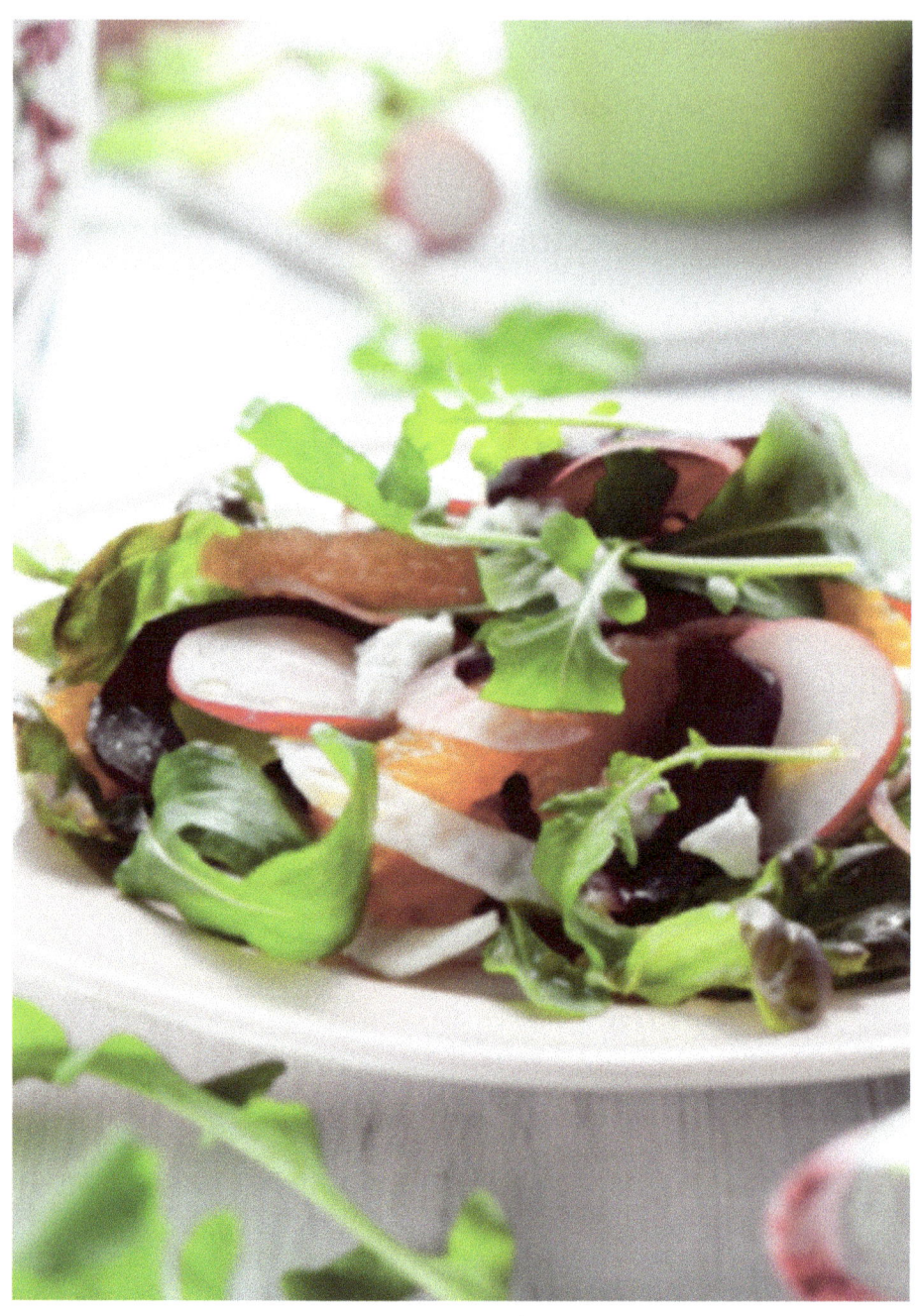

Potato rosti with beetroot horseradish

Ingredients

- 1½ teaspoons of cumin seeds
- 2 medium beetroots
- ½ a red onion
- 2 tablespoons of creamed horseradish
- 1 clove of garlic
- 2 large potatoes
- 3 tablespoons of vegetable oil

Directions

- Coarsely grate and squeeze out excess liquid from the potatoes.
- Then, combine the potatoes together with the onion, toasted cumin, and garlic in a large bowl, season.
- Shape into 4 patties with your hands.
- Heat olive oil in a pan.
- Fry the rosti over a medium-low heat for 10 minutes on each side, turning carefully.

- Combine the grated beetroot with horseradish in a bowl and serve on top of the rosti.
- Enjoy.

Beetroot nicoise salad

Ingredients

- 1 bunch of fresh mixed soft herbs
- 2 small cos lettuce
- 4 slices of sourdough bread
- 12 quail eggs
- 500g of raw mixed baby beetroots
- 1 tablespoon of red wine vinegar
- 2 teaspoons of Dijon mustard
- 1 tablespoon of baby capers
- 4 salted anchovy fillets
- 4 tablespoons of extra virgin olive oil
- 150g of fine French beans
- 100g of ripe cherry tomatoes

Directions

- Boil water in large pans.
- Place beetroots into one of the pans, keeping some for later, let boil for 10 minutes. Slice the reserved beets.
- Whisking extra virgin olive oil with vinegar, mustard, and capers.

- Season with sea salt and black pepper.
- Drain the beetroots in a colander and steam dry.
- Peel the skin and slice any larger beetroots in half.
- Transfer the beetroots to a bowl, drizzle over half the dressing, toss to coat.
- In the other pan, add the quail eggs with the French beans, let simmer for 4 minutes, then drain.
- Add the flavoring herbs to the leftover dressing, place into a salad bowl.
- Layer up the tomatoes in the salad bowl with the lettuce and anchovies, drizzle over the dressing.
- Next, tumble in the cooked and raw beetroots with the eggs and green beans.
- Scatter over the remaining herbs.
- Serve and enjoy with the sourdough.

Beetroot crisp with coriander hummus

Ingredients

- 1 teaspoon of smoked paprika
- 250g of large beetroot
- 1 lemon
- 3 sprigs of fresh thyme
- 2 tablespoons of tahini
- Olive oil
- Extra virgin olive oil
- 2 cloves of garlic
- 1 x 400g tin of chickpeas
- 50g of coriander leaves

Directions

- Preheat your oven ready to 400°F.
- Place sliced beetroots in a bowl. Toss in the thyme leaves with bit of olive oil.
- Spread on a lined baking trays, let roast for 15 minutes, let cool.
- In a blender, crush the garlic, and pour in the chickpeas with their juices.

- Add the remaining ingredients with bit of extra virgin olive oil, blend until smooth.
- Season, drizzle with extra virgin olive oil in a bowl.
- Serve and enjoy.

Roasted beetroot, red onion, and watercress salad

Ingredients

- 5 tablespoons of olive oil
- 3 tablespoons of baby caper
- 2 x 600g bunches of beetroot
- 4 red onions
- 125ml of white wine
- A few sprigs of fresh dill
- 4 tablespoons of extra virgin olive oil
- A few sprigs of fresh mint leaves
- 4 cloves of garlic
- A few sprigs of parsley leaves
- 2 x 75g bags of watercress
- 3 tablespoons of balsamic vinegar
- 1 tablespoon of Dijon mustard

Directions

- Preheat the oven to 340°F.
- Place sliced beetroots in a baking tin with 2 tablespoons of olive oil, fill the tin with water.
- Cover the dish with tin foil, let bake for 1 hour.
- Remove the beets from the tin, let cool.
- Toss the onion wedges in 2 tablespoons of the olive oil on the baking tray, season.
- Add to the oven, let roast for about 30 minutes.
- Remove, let cool.
- Rub the off the beetroot skins, cut into wedges.
- Blanch the beetroot stalks and leaves in a pan of boiling salted water for 2 minutes, drain.
- Heat the remaining tablespoon of oil in a pan over a high heat.
- Then, add the beetroot stalks and garlic and fry until the garlic is golden.
- Lower the heat to medium, pour in the wine, let cook for 10 minutes.
- Add the beetroot leaves, season, cook until wilted.

- Whisk the vinegar into the mustard, then stir in the olive oil and season to taste.
- In a large serving bowl, gently toss the roasted beetroot and red onions with the stalk mixture, chopped herbs, capers and vinaigrette, then mix with the watercress.
- Serve and enjoy.

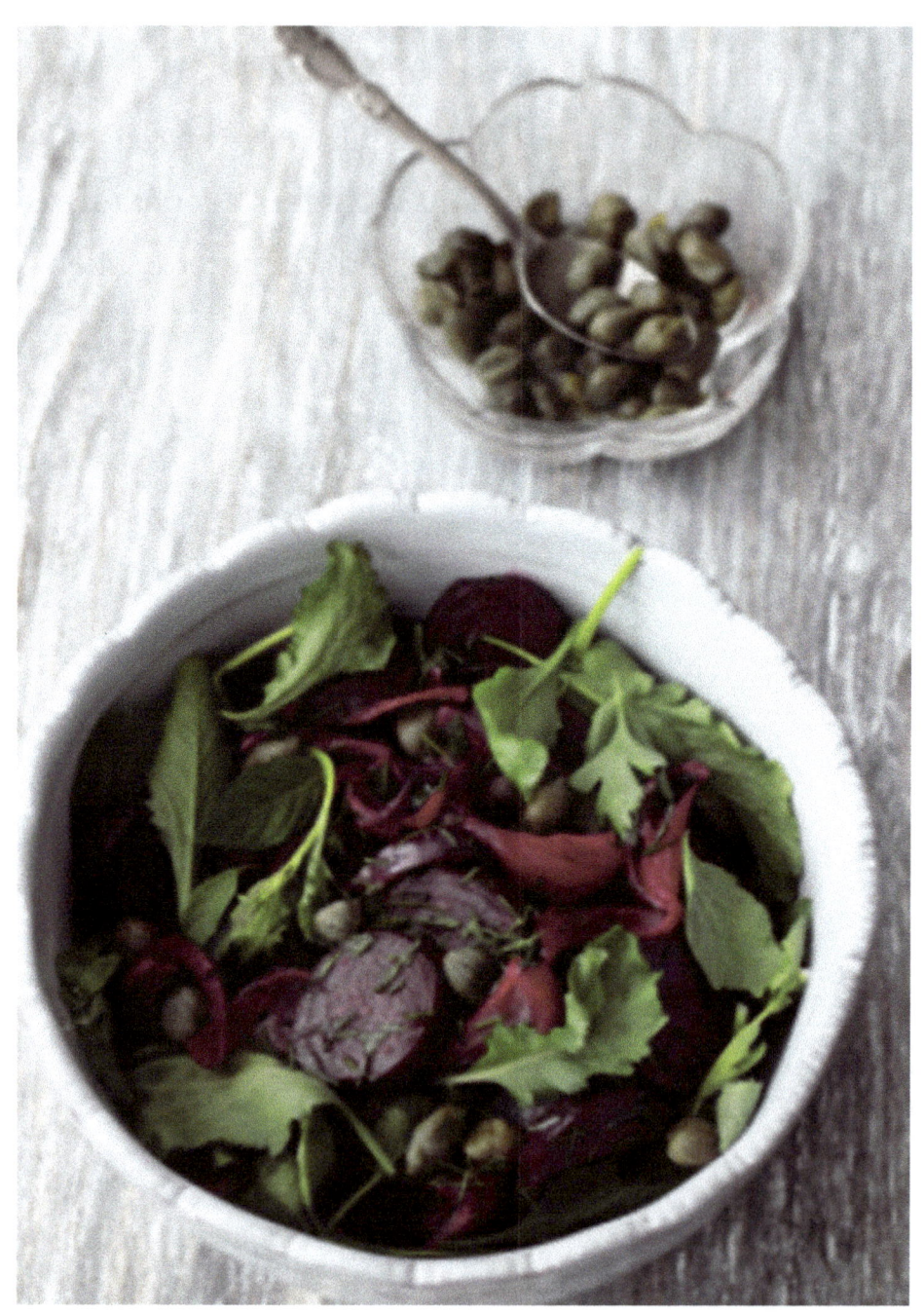

Harvest salad

Ingredients

- 2 tablespoon of red wine vinegar
- 6 tablespoons of extra virgin olive oil
- 6 small beetroots
- 1 red onion
- 2 bulbs of fennel
- 1 teaspoon of Dijon mustard
- Olive oil
- 2 teaspoons of coriander seeds
- ½ a bunch of fresh mint
- 1 acorn squash
- ½ a bunch of fresh flat-leaf parsley
- 1 pomegranate
- 150g of feta cheese

Directions

- Preheat the oven ready to 380°F.
- Lay cut squash pieces, beetroots, fennel wedges and sliced onions in a roasting tray.
- Drizzle with a little olive oil.

- Pound the coriander seeds with a good pinch each of sea salt and black pepper.
- Sprinkle over the vegetables on the tray, toss to coat.
- Let roast for about 40 minutes, shaking halfway through. Let cool slightly.
- The, combine the vinegar together with the extra virgin olive oil, mustard, and seasoning in a small jug. Mix well.
- Dress the roasted veg while still warm so they soak up all the dressing.
- Sprinkle over the herb leaves, and reserved fennel tops.
- Add the pomegranate to the vegetables. Crumble over the feta.
- Serve and enjoy.

Roasted beetroot toast

Ingredients

- 4 slices of sourdough
- A few fresh chives
- 4 tablespoons of red wine vinegar
- 4 raw beetroots
- 5 sprigs of fresh thyme
- 2 tablespoons of creamed horseradish

Directions

- Preheat the oven to 350°F.
- Place wedges of beetroot in a roasting tray.
- Add the vinegar together with the thyme and 4 tablespoons of water, toss to coat.
- Cover with tin foil, then let roast for 45 minutes.
- Toast the bread and spread with the horseradish topping with the roasted beetroot.
- Serve and enjoy.

Warm potato, herring, beetroot and apple salad

Ingredients

- 4 tablespoons of olive oil
- 200g of beetroot
- 2 tablespoons of red wine vinegar
- 1 pinch of granulated sugar
- 500g of Ratte potatoes
- A few fresh chives
- 1 small apple
- 1 lug of sparkling water
- 2 marinated herring fillets
- ½ tablespoon of Dijon mustard

Directions

- For the vinaigrette, combine the Dijon mustard together with the olive oil, red wine vinegar, and sugar in a bowl.
- Season with sea salt and black pepper, then whisk to blend.
- Add the sparkling water to loosen the mixture, then whisk.

- Cook the beetroot in a pan of boiling salted water for 45 minutes.
- In another separate pan of boiling salted water, cook unpeeled potatoes for 20 minutes. Drain in a colander, then slice warm.
- Drain and allow the beetroot to cool slightly, then slice.
- Divide the potato, beetroot, apple slices and herring fillets among 4 serving plates.
- Drizzle over the vinaigrette, chop and scatter over the chives.
- Serve and enjoy with warm potatoes.

Beetroot dip

Ingredients

- 4 vac-packed beetroot
- 1 tablespoon of horseradish
- Rye bread
- 1 teaspoon of caraway seeds
- 3 sprigs of fresh thyme
- 3 tablespoons of crème fraiche

Directions

- Pick the thyme leaves, and blend all the ingredients in a food processor.
- Season with sea salt and black pepper.
- Serve and enjoy with rye bread.

Beetroot, almond, and ricotta

Ingredients

- 2 tablespoons of ground almonds
- 2 tablespoons of ricotta cheese
- Vac-packed cooked beetroot

Directions

- Place the beetroot in a blender.
- Add the ground almonds together with the ricotta cheese to the blender, a purée.
- Adjust thickness with water.
- Serve and enjoy.

Chili pickled sweet and sour beets

Ingredients

- 3 fresh red chillies
- 100ml of balsamic vinegar
- 1 tablespoon coriander seeds
- 400ml of white wine vinegar
- 200g of golden caster sugar
- 1/2 lemon
- 1.5 kg of beetroots

Directions

- Place the beets in a pan of salted water and bring to the boil.
- Let simmer for 30 minutes until cooked, then drain. Let cool.
- Add the vinegars together with the sugar in a separate pan.
- Add halved chilies to the pan with a squeeze of lemon juice, coriander seeds, and a pinch of sea salt, over a high heat.
- Bring to the boil, stirring until the sugar is dissolved.

- Spoon the beets into jars, pour the pickling liquid on top.
- Add a chili to each jar, seal, infuse for few days
- Serve and enjoy.

Beetroot, peach, and coconut no cook recipe

Ingredients

- 100 ml of coconut milk
- 1 whole ripe peach
- 1 vac-packed cooked beetroot

Directions

- Place peeled peach in a blender.
- Add the beetroot.
- Pour in the coconut milk, blend until smooth.
- Adjust its thickness with water.
- Serve and enjoy.

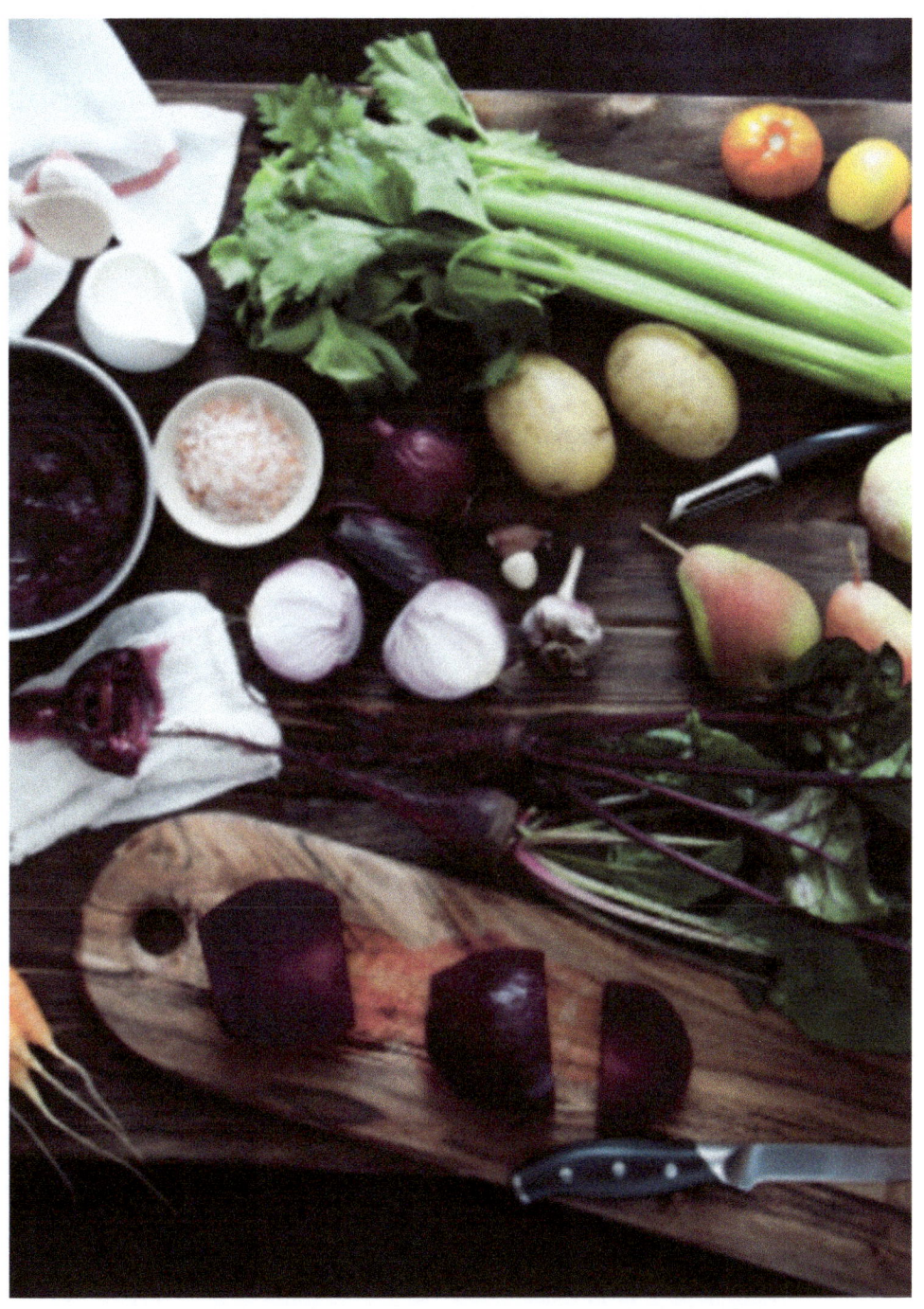

Pink risotto

Ingredients

- ½ x 220g tin of chopped tomatoes
- ½ of a small onion
- 50g of basmati rice
- 2 vac-packed beetroot
- ½ tablespoon of olive oil

Directions

- Heat the olive oil in a medium pan over medium heat.
- Add the onions, let fry for 5 minutes.
- Then, add the rice stirring until well coated.
- Pour in boiling water, cook for 8 minutes covered.
- Stir in the beetroot together with the tomatoes.
- Lower the heat, let cook until all the liquid has been absorbed.
- Then, mash until fairly smooth, with some soft lumps.
- Serve and enjoy.

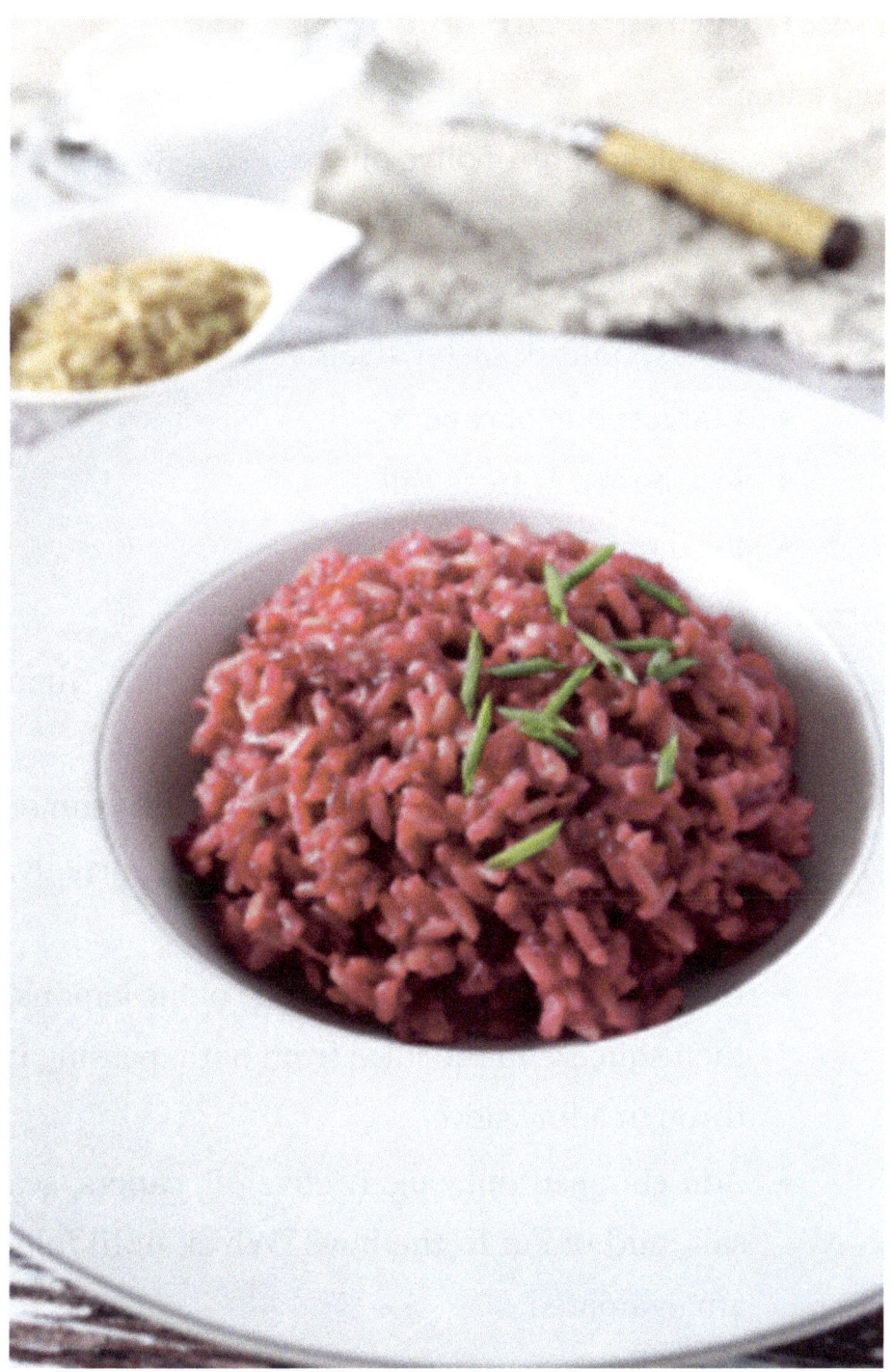

Vegan beetroot carpaccio

Ingredients

- 2 tablespoons of olive oil
- 8 medium beetroots
- 2 lemons
- 2 teaspoons of caster sugar
- 1 tablespoon of capers
- ½ a bunch of fresh dill
- 1 red onion

Directions

- Place the beetroot in a large saucepan, then cover with water.
- Bring to the boil, lower the heat, let simmer gently, for 40 minutes, covered partially. Drain and set aside.
- Into a bowl, grate the zest of one of the lemons, then squeeze in the juice from both, passing it through a fine sieve.
- Add chopped dill, sugar, olive oil, capers, sea salt, and onion to the bowl. Whisk until fully amalgamated.

- Run the beetroots under a cold tap and gently slide off the skins.
- Then, slice the beetroot into thin rounds.
- Arrange the beetroot slices on a serving platter.
- Spoon over the dressing, allow it to sink into the crevice of the beetroots.
- Then, cover with Clingfilm, place in the fridge for 4 hours.
- Remove, serve and enjoy.

Candied beet salad

Ingredients

- 75ml of buttermilk
- 750g of golden beetroot
- 150g of golden caster sugar
- Juice of 1 lemon
- 50g of mixed seeds
- Extra virgin olive oil
- 1/2 teaspoon of sweet smoked paprika
- 1/2 bunch of mixed soft herbs
- 2 knobs of unsalted butter
- Zest and juice of 1 orange
- 1/4 teaspoon of ground cinnamon
- 2 handfuls of salad leaves

Directions

- Place the beets in water, bring to the boil over a high heat, reduce heat let simmer and cook for 1 hour.
- Drain, let cool. then, peel off the skins and roughly cut into 3cm wedges.

- Toss the seeds in a little olive oil with the paprika and a pinch of sea salt and black pepper.
- Toast in a dry frying pan until golden.
- Whisk the buttermilk in a jug together with the juice of half the lemon, and olive oil. Season.
- Stir into the dressing chopped herbs, place to one side.
- Melt the butter in the same frying pan used for toasting the seeds.
- Finely grate in the zest of the orange.
- Add a squeeze of orange juice together with the cinnamon, sugar, and a pinch of salt and pepper.
- Bring to the boil and leave to bubble away for 10 minutes.
- Remove from the heat and toss through the cooked beets.
- Toss the salad leaves with the buttermilk dressing and scatter over the beets.
- Serve and enjoy with the toasted seeds.

Rainbow salad wrap

Ingredients

- 3 teaspoons of cider vinegar
- 2 small raw beetroots
- 50g of feta cheese
- 2 carrots
- 5 tablespoons of natural yogurt
- 150g of white cabbage
- 2 tablespoons of extra virgin olive oil
- 1 pear
- ½ a bunch of fresh mint
- ½ teaspoon of English mustard
- ½ a bunch of parsley
- 6 small whole meal tortilla wraps

Directions

- Firstly, place the grated carrots, cabbage, pear, mint, parsley leaves, and beetroots into a large bowl.
- Add natural yogurt, English mustard, cider vinegar, and extra virgin olive oil to a jam jar.
- Secure the lid and shake well.

- Taste and adjust accordingly.
- Drizzle most of the dressing over the salad.
- Divide the salad between the tortilla wraps, crumble a little feta over each.
- Roll up the wraps, tucking them in at the sides.
- Serve and enjoy.

Mandolin salad

Ingredients

- ½ Bunch of fresh mint
- 50ml of milk
- 3 large raw beetroots
- Rapeseed oil
- 2 apples
- 200g of soft goat's cheese
- Cider vinegar

Directions

- Begin by whisking the goat's cheese together with the milk in a food processor until blended with a thick cream.
- Season with sea salt and black pepper.
- Spoon over a large platter.
- Toss sliced beets and apples together with a little drizzle of olive oil and a tiny splash of cider vinegar.
- Pile it all on top of the goat's cheese mix.
- Sprinkle sliced mint over.
- Serve and enjoy immediately.

Gorgeous roast vegetables

Ingredients

- Sea salt
- 800g of mixed-color carrot
- Freshly ground black pepper
- 800g of potatoes
- 350g of parsnips
- 6 tablespoon of duck fat
- 350g of raw beetroot
- A few sprigs of fresh rosemary

Directions

- Start by dividing the vegetables between a few large pans, cover with boiling salted water and parboil for 15 minutes.
- Drain in a large colander, steam dry for some minutes.
- Shake the colander to chuff up the edges, place in the largest roasting tray.
- Drizzle with the duck fat, put the rosemary leaves over.
- Season with salt and pepper, toss to coat.

- Push the vegetables into a single layer.
- At 425°F, cook for 40 minutes or so, turning halfway through.
- Serve and enjoy with the roast duck.

Root vegetable salad

Ingredients

- Freshly ground black pepper
- Sea salt
- 3 carrots
- 3 raw beetroots
- 1 fennel bulb
- 5 tablespoons of extra virgin olive oil
- 1 bunch of radishes
- 1 celery heart
- ½ a bunch of fresh mint
- ½ a small radicchio
- 1 lemon

Directions

- Place the carrots with beetroots, radishes, celery, lettuce, fennel bulbs in a large mixing bowl.
- Squeeze lemon juice into a small bowl, add mind leaves with extra virgin olive oil.
- Whisk together with a fork, then shake well.

- Taste the dressing, adjust the season with a tiny pinch of salt and pepper.
- Pour over the root vegetables.
- Toss the vegetables in the dressing.
- Transfer to a serving bowl and sprinkle over the fennel tops and reserved baby mint.
- Serve and enjoy.

Home-cured beetroot gravadlax

Ingredients

- 1 loaf of brown bread
- 2 large fresh beetroots
- A few handfuls of watercress
- 50ml of gin
- 1 orange
- 2 lemons
- 2 juniper berries
- 1 lemon, cut into wedges
- 6 tablespoons of rock salt
- 1 small bunch fresh tarragon
- 2 tablespoons of demerara sugar
- 50ml of gin
- 800g of side of salmon
- 1 small bunch fresh dill
- 4 tablespoons of freshly grated horseradish

Directions

- Blend the beetroots together with the orange, lemon zest, and juniper berries in a food processor until fairly smooth paste forms.

- Transfer this to a bowl and stir in the rock salt and sugar.
- Pour in the gin and mix.
- Lay the salmon with the skin-side down on a large baking tray.
- Gently pour over the beetroot cure.
- Spread all over the salmon flesh in a uniform manner.
- Then, wrap the salmon in a double layer of greaseproof paper, wrap with Clingfilm.
- Refrigerate for 24 hours.
- Take the salmon out of the fridge, unwrap to rinse off the cure.
- Push the beetroot cure off the fish.
- Place the rinsed salmon to one side and run the tray under the tap.
- Mix together the chopped herbs, horseradish, and gin.
- Put the salmon back into the clean tray, skin-side down.
- Pack the herby cure onto the salmon using your hands.

- Wrap with a double layer of greaseproof paper, refrigerate for 24 hours.
- The following day your salmon will be perfectly cured and ready to eat.
- Serve and enjoy.

Roasted vegetable mega mix

Ingredients

- 5 fresh bay leaves
- 2 bulbs of fennel
- Olive oil
- 350g of beetroot
- A few sprigs of fresh thyme
- 2 balsamic vinegar
- A few sprigs of fresh oregano
- White wine vinegar
- 500g of carrots
- 1 clementine
- A few sprigs of fresh rosemary
- 400g of parsnips
- ½ of a lemon
- 3 sprigs of fresh sage
- 1 small teaspoon of runny honey
- 350g of baby turnips
- 2 of red wine vinegar

Directions

- Preheat your oven to 375°F.

- Bring two large pans of salted water to the boil.
- Place beets in one of the pans, keep separated from the rest of the vegetables. Boil for 25 minutes or so.
- Place carrots, parsnips, and fennel in the second pan, boil for 10 minutes.
- Drain, let steam dry, then separate to hit them with those different flavors.
- Toss the beets with the balsamic vinegar and whole herb sprigs.
- Toss the carrots with the clementine juice, place in the squeezed halves, pick over the rosemary leaves.
- Toss the parsnips with the vinegar and tear over the sage leaves.
- Toss the turnips with the vinegar and bay.
- Toss the fennel with the lemon juice, place over the thyme leaves.
- Lay them out on a large tray, according to veggie types.
- Let roast until golden and crispy.

- Drizzle with the honey over the parsnips the veggies are about to get ready.
- Serve and enjoy.

Rainbow trout with horseradish yogurt and balsamic beets

Ingredients

- 4 jarred beetroots
- 400g of potatoes
- 1 heaped teaspoon of creamed horseradish
- Balsamic vinegar
- Sea salt
- 2 handfuls of watercress
- Freshly ground black pepper
- 4 x 100g of rainbow trout fillets
- Extra virgin olive oil
- 2 heaped tablespoons of natural yoghurt
- Olive oil
- A few sprigs fresh thyme
- 1 lemon

Directions

- Add the potatoes to a pan of salted boiling water, let cook for 15 minutes.
- Put a large frying pan on a medium heat.

- Then, season the trout on both sides with a pinch of salt and pepper.
- Add olive oil to the pan, scatter in the thyme tips, trout.
- Press down on the fish to crisp up the skin, let cook for 4 minutes.
- In a small bowl, mix the yoghurt together with the juice of ½ a lemon, horseradish, and a small pinch of salt.
- Dress the beets with a splash of balsamic and a small pinch of salt.
- Drain the potatoes, toss with a pinch of salt and pepper and a drizzle of olive oil.
- Serve and enjoy with a dollop of yogurt, radish, and drizzle of extra virgin olive oil.

Raw beetroot salad

Ingredients

- Fresh horseradish
- Pepper
- Beetroots
- Salt
- Flat-leaf parsley

Directions

- Combine sliced beets with flavors, chopped parsley leaves, salt, pepper, and grated horseradish.
- Let rest for 10 minutes to allow the horseradish to soften the beetroot.
- Toss with a splash of vodka.
- Serve and enjoy.

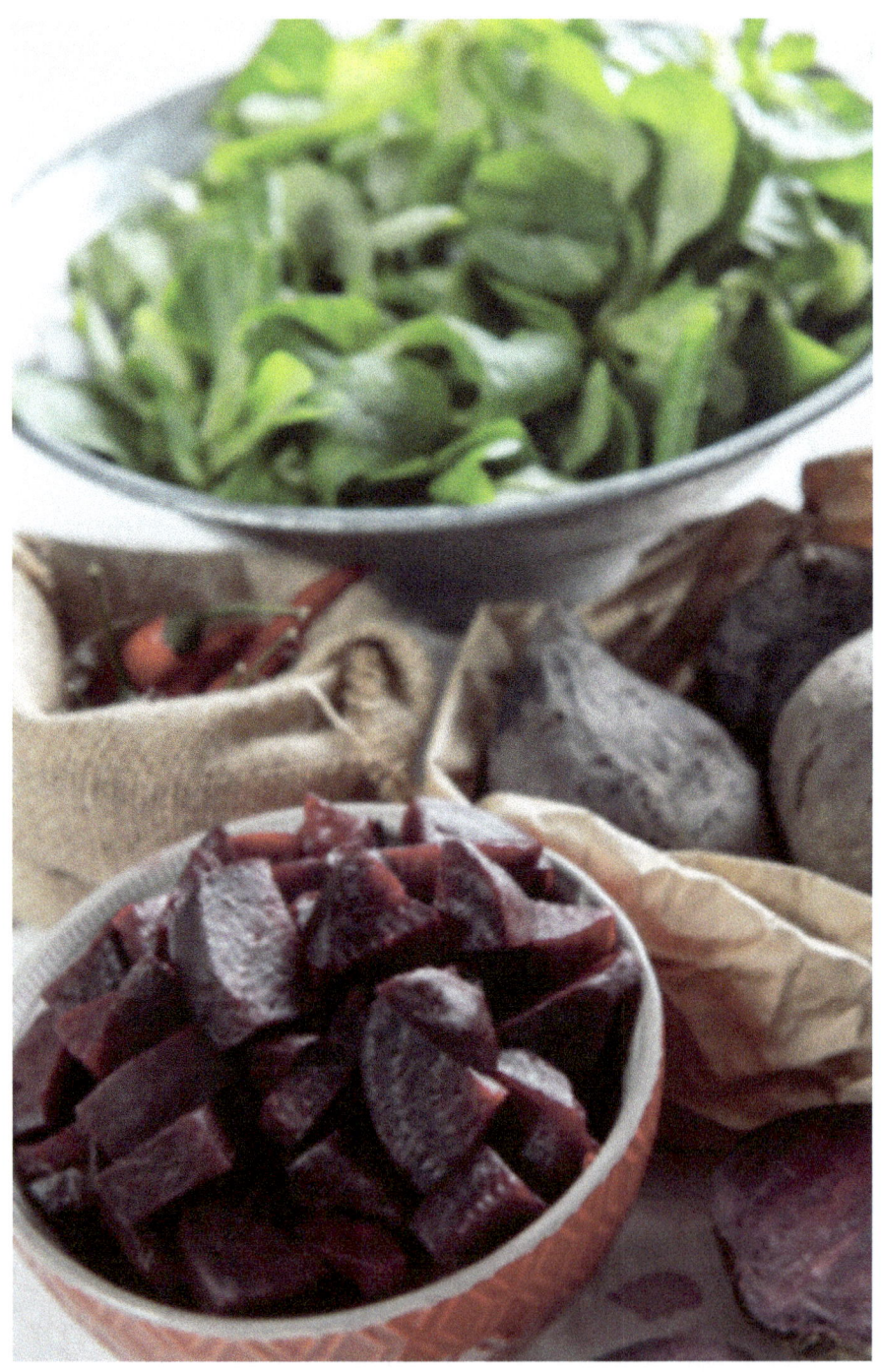

Fresh smoked salmon and beetroot salad

Ingredients

- Balsamic vinegar
- 4 raw baby beetroot
- 2cm piece of fresh horseradish
- ½ lemon
- Sea salt
- Freshly ground black pepper
- 1 loaf of granary bread
- Extra virgin olive oil
- 200g of smoked salmon
- 35g of watercress

Directions

- Begin by shaving the beetroot into a bowl.
- Then, add the lemon juice with a small pinch of salt and pepper, extra virgin olive oil, and a splash of balsamic vinegar, mix well
- Organize the smoked salmon in waves over a large platter.

- Then, Scatter over the watercress, then the beetroot slices, leaving any juices behind in the bowl.
- Over the beetroot, grate the horseradish, then spoon the juices from the beetroot over the top.
- Sprinkle with an extra pinch of pepper and a drizzle of extra virgin olive oil.
- Serve and enjoy with fresh loaf of granary bread.

Crunchy raw beetroot salad with feta and pear

Ingredients

- 1 lemon
- 3 ripe pears
- Extra virgin olive oil
- 4 large beetroot
- A few sprigs of fresh mint
- 1 large handful of sunflower seeds
- 200g of feta cheese

Directions

- Squeeze the lemon juice into a clean jam jar.
- Top with 10 tablespoons of oil, and a pinch of sea salt and black pepper.
- Shake the jar once the lid is secured, keep aside until needed.
- Dress the matchsticks in a little of the lemon oil dressing.
- Taste, and adjust the flavors and seasoning.
- Divide the salad between plates, crumble over the creamy feta.

- Sprinkle chopped mint leaves over the salad with the sunflower seeds.
- Serve and enjoy.

Beetroot, red apple, and watercress salad

Ingredients

- 1 small handful of pea shoots
- 2 small red beetroot
- ½ a bunch of fresh marjoram
- 2 small candy beetroot
- 2 red eating apples
- ½ of a lemon
- extra virgin olive oil
- 1 bag of rocket
- 40g of watercress

Directions

- Squeeze the lemon juice into a clean jam jar.
- Add three times the amount of extra virgin olive oil.
- Then, season with sea salt and black pepper.
- Fasten or secure the lid and shake to emulsify.
- Add the rocket together with the watercress, pea shoots, beetroot, and apples to a large bowl.

- Drizzle over enough dressing to coat the ingredients.
- Place in the marjoram leaves, toss again.
- Serve and enjoy.

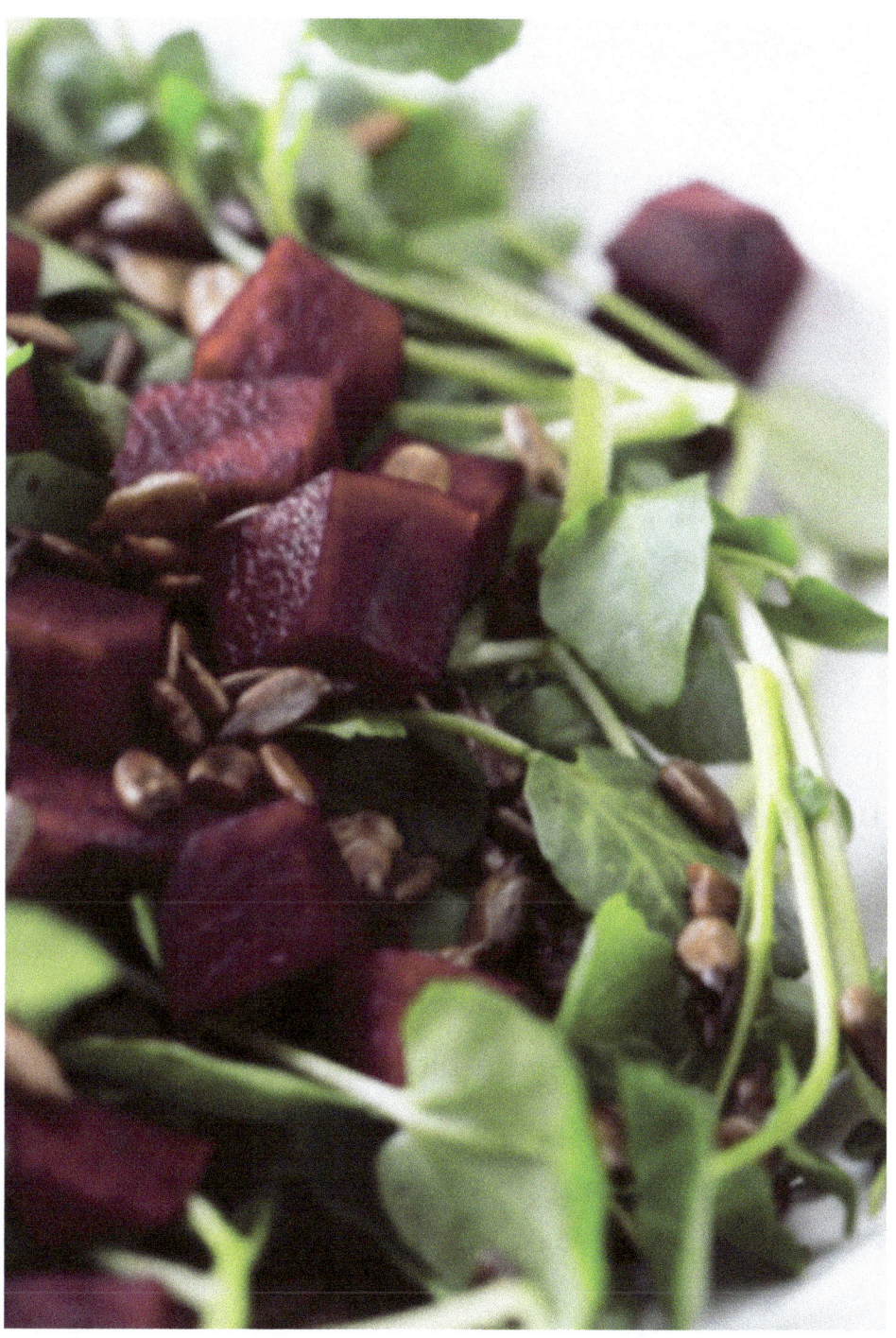

Avocado pastry quiche

Ingredients

- 2 ripe avocados
- 100g bag of mixed salad
- Extra virgin olive oil
- 400g of self-raising flour
- 1 lemon
- Olive oil
- 6 large free-range eggs
- 300g of frozen peas
- 90g of cheddar cheese
- ½ a bunch of basil

Directions

- Preheat the oven to 400°F
- In a large bowl, smash up the avocado, then rub in the flour with a pinch of sea salt and 4 tablespoons of cold water until it foams a dough.
- Knead until smooth.
- Wrap and rest for 15 minutes.

- Crack the eggs into a blender, add the frozen peas and most of the Cheddar.
- Place basil leaves with a pinch of salt and black pepper, blend until smooth.
- Roll out the avocado pastry on a flour-dusted surface.
- Loosely roll it up around the rolling pin, then unroll it over an oiled baking tray.
- Let bake for 10 minutes, or until lightly golden.
- Pour in the filling and bake for another 15 minutes.
- Dress the salad leaves with extra virgin olive oil and lemon juice.
- Season, and sprinkle over the quiche.
- Serve and enjoy.

Fluffy flourless pancake

Ingredients

- 2 large free-range eggs
- Chili sauce
- 2 large free-range eggs
- 100g of porridge oats
- 1 teaspoon of baking powder
- Olive oil
- 100g of cottage cheese
- 1 avocado

Directions

- Put the oats together with the cottage cheese, 2 eggs, and the baking powder in a blender, process until smooth with a tiny pinch of sea salt.
- Heat a large non-stick frying pan over a medium-high heat with a small splash of oil.
- Add the batter to the pan, little by little at a time.
- Let fry for 2 minutes, or until golden, flipping halfway.

- Serve and enjoy topping with sliced avocado, a fried egg and chili sauce.

Roasted black beans burgers

This incredible fruity recipe features mangos and tabasco with beans and zingy tomato perfect for a Mediterranean Sea diet.

Ingredients

- 1 ripe avocado
- 200g of mixed mushrooms
- 4 tablespoons of natural yoghurt
- 100g of rye bread
- Chipotle tabasco sauce
- Ground coriander
- 1 x 400g tin of black beans
- 4 sprigs of fresh coriander
- 1 lime
- Olive oil
- 40g of mature cheddar cheese
- 1 ripe mango
- 1½ red onions
- 4 soft rolls
- 100g of ripe cherry tomatoes

Directions

- First, preheat the oven ready to 400°F.
- Combine onion, rye bread, mushroom, and 1 teaspoon of coriander in a food processor, blend until fine.
- Drain and pulse in the black beans.
- Then, season lightly with sea salt and black pepper.
- Divide into 4 and shape into patties.
- Rub all over with oil and dust with ground coriander.
- Transfer to an oiled baking tray, let roast for 25 minutes, or until dark.
- Place remaining chopped onion, tomato in a bowl.
- Then, squeeze over the lime juice, with few shakes of Tabasco and season to taste.
- Halve the warm rolls and divide the yoghurt between the bases, with salsa, mango, avocado, and coriander leaves.
- Top with the burgers, remaining salsa and extra Tabasco.

- Serve and enjoy.

Mexican baked eggs

Ingredients

- ½ a lime
- 4 large free-range eggs
- 1 red chili
- Olive oil
- 2 sprigs of fresh coriander
- 1 ripe avocado

Directions

- Preheat the oven to high hot.
- Then, grease a small skillet pan with a drizzle of olive oil, crack in the eggs.
- Scatter sliced red chili over the eggs.
- juice of one half.
- Organize the avocado around the eggs.
- Season with a little sea salt and black pepper.
- Place in the oven for 10 minutes, or until the egg whites are set.
- Sprinkle some coriander leaves over the eggs.
- Cut the remaining lime into wedges, squeeze over.

- Serve and enjoy with hot buttered toast.

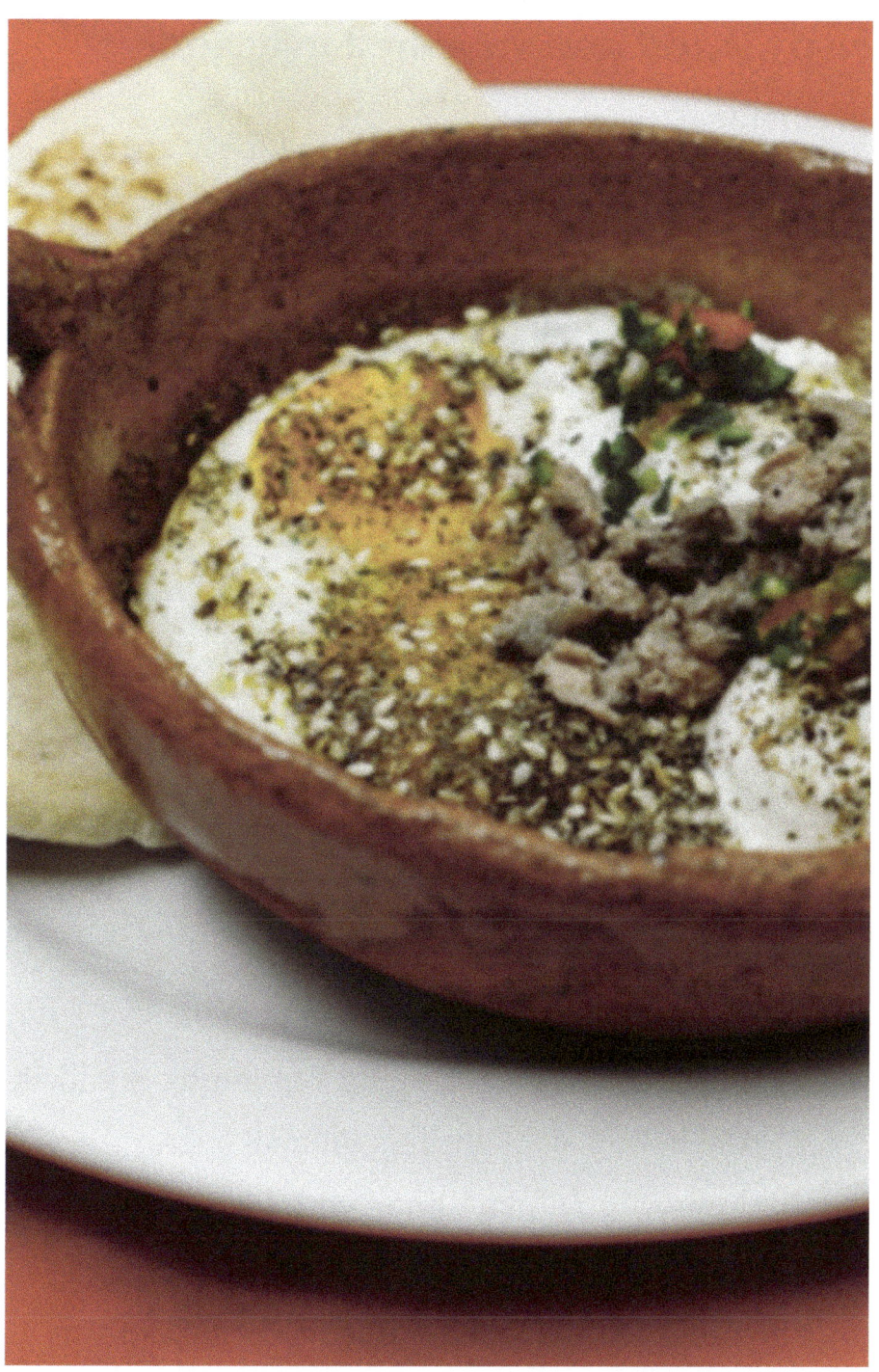

Crispy squid and smashed avocado

Ingredients

- 2 limes
- 2 heaped tablespoons of whole meal flour
- 1 ripe avocado
- 2 teaspoons of hot chili sauce
- 250g of squid, gutted, cleaned

Directions

- Pour olive oil into a large frying pan on a medium-high heat, let heat up.
- Toss all the squid with the flour and a pinch of sea salt and black pepper to coat.
- Scoop the avocado flesh into a bowl.
- Grate in the zest of 1 lime, squeeze in the juice and mash until smooth.
- Taste, an adjust the seasoning.
- Piece by piece, place the remaining squid in the hot oil, cook until golden all over.
- Remove to a plate lined with kitchen paper to drain excess olive oil.

- Drizzle over the chili sauce and a little extra virgin olive oil.
- Serve and enjoy with lime wedges.

Avocado on rye toast with ricotta

Ingredients

- 1 teaspoon of toasted pine nuts
- 1 ripe tomato
- 1 heaped teaspoon of ricotta cheese
- 1 lemon
- 1 sprig of fresh basil
- 1 x 75g slice of rye bread
- ½ of a ripe avocado

Directions

- Begin by spreading the ricotta cheese over the rye bread.
- Then, slice the avocado with tomato,
- Toss with a squeeze of lemon juice.
- Season accordingly and arrange on the toast.
- Sprinkle over the pine nuts and a few fresh baby basil leaves.
- Serve and enjoy.

Avocado on rye toast with chocolate

Ingredients

- Raspberries
- ½ of a ripe avocado
- Dark chocolate
- ½ of a ripe banana
- 1 x 75g slice of rye bread
- 1 heaped teaspoon of light cream cheese
- 2 teaspoons of toasted hazelnuts
- 1 teaspoon of cocoa powder

Directions

- Smash up the avocado together with the banana, cream cheese, and cocoa powder until smooth.
- Spread over the rye bread.
- Dot over a few raspberries with the toasted hazelnuts.
- Shave over a tiny bit of dark chocolate.
- Serve and enjoy.

Mega veggie nachos

This is a favorite for most vegetarians and other Mediterranean Sea diet lovers. It features variety of fruits and vegetables along with herbs for a perfect taste and flavor.

Ingredients

- 1 ripe avocado
- 1 fresh red chili
- 1 x 400g tin of black beans
- 3 ripe tomatoes
- 20g of feta cheese
- 6 spring onions
- 1 bunch of fresh coriander
- 2 limes
- 2 mixed-color peppers
- Chipotle Tabasco sauce
- Extra virgin olive oil
- 4 corn tortillas
- ½ teaspoon of cumin seeds

Directions

- Place the oven on to 350°F.

- Place a griddle pan over a high heat and cook the whole peppers, together with chili, tomatoes, and trimmed spring onions until charred.
- Place the peppers and chili in a bowl, cover with Clingfilm, set aside briefly.
- Combine tomatoes, spring onions, peppers, and chilies in a bowl.
- Season few coriander leaves, then mix in a squeeze of lime juice and a drizzle of oil.
- Cut the tortillas into wedges and arrange over the baking sheets.
- Let bake for 5 minutes and or until golden.
- Toast the cumin seeds over high heat.
- Add the Tabasco sauce with beans, cook for a few minutes, stirring occasionally.
- Drizzle avocado wedges with the remaining lime juice.
- Arrange the tortillas in a bowl.
- Top with the beans, salsa, dressed avocado, feta.
- Serve and enjoy.

Avocado on rye toast with beetroot

Ingredients

- ½ of a ripe avocado
- 1 beetroot
- 1 teaspoon of extra virgin olive oil
- 1 teaspoon of mixed seeds
- 1 teaspoon of hummus
- 1 teaspoon of cottage cheese
- 1 x 75g of slice of rye bread

Directions

- Start by smashing up the beetroot together with the hummus and cottage cheese.
- Season to taste and spread over the rye bread.
- Place ripe avocado on top.
- Drizzle with the extra virgin olive oil.
- Sprinkle with mixed seeds.
- Serve and enjoy.

Baked sweet potatoes, avocado, and queso fresco

Ingredients

- 150g of Mexican queso fresco
- 4 sweet potatoes
- 2 limes
- Olive oil
- 1 handful of pumpkin seeds
- 2 ripe avocados

Directions

- Preheat the oven ready to 380°F.
- Drizzle the potatoes with oil.
- Season with a sprinkle of sea salt and black pepper.
- Wrap in a foil and bake in the oven for 1 hour and 15 minutes.
- When the potatoes are nearly done, destone and roughly chop the avocados and toss with the juice from half a lime.
- Toast the pumpkin seeds in a dry pan briefly until slightly golden.

- Top the potatoes with the avocado, then crumble over the cheese.
- Sprinkle with the toasted seeds.
- Serve and enjoy with lime wedges.